The Issue of Blood
&
Living with Fibroids

RENITA LEWIS

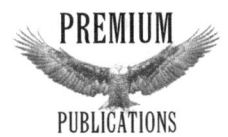

Copyright © 2016 by Renita Lewis
All Rights Reserved

THE ISSUE OF BLOOD & LIVING WITH FIBROIDS
by Renita Lewis

Published by PREMIUM PUBLICATIONS
PO Box 1555
Bonita Springs, FL. 34133
www.premiumpublications.org

Printed in the United States of America

This book or parts thereof may not be used or reproduced in any form, stored in a retrieval system, or transmitted in any form by any means electronic, mechanical, photocopy, recording or otherwise without prior written permission of the publisher, except as provided by United States of America copyright law.

All Scripture quotations, unless otherwise indicated, are taken from the Amplified Bible, Copyright © 1954, 1958, 1962, 1964, 1965, 1987 by The Lockman Foundation. Used by permission.

First Edition
Cover Design/layout by Delaney-Designs.com

Library of Congress Control Number: 2 0 1 6 9 4 5 8 1 4
ISBN: 978-0-9977451-0-8

This book is dedicated to every woman who suffers with fibroids or the issue of blood.

My hope is to bring knowledge and understanding to people all over the world about the pain, suffering, humiliation, and the associated cost that many women experience who suffers with fibroids or the issue of blood.

TABLE OF CONTENT

Introduction 7
Isolation 9
Shame 17
Helpless 23
Lord Please Keep My Mind Through It All 27
Emotions 33
Help I am Anemic 39
No Health Insurance 45
The Beast Within 53
Blood 59
Vaginal Discharge 65
The Womb 71
The Pain of it All 77
When you have done all that you know to do 81
Surgery 87
All is Well 93

Introduction

I didn't write this book to discuss the next cure for fibroids. I would like to share my personal journey along with some of my pain and suffering that I have experienced while living with fibroids and the issue of blood. If you are a woman who is currently living with fibroids or the issue of blood then you will be able to identify with some of my experiences that I will openly talk about. Many women who are living with fibroids are scared to talk about the shame, humiliation, cost, fear and emotional distress that come along with living with fibroids or the issue of blood. The purpose of this book is to encourage women all over the world by sharing my own personal experience. What is written in this book is not the experience of every woman who has fibroids or the issue of blood. It's for women, like me who had moments where they wished they were dead. "At least those were some of my moments". Living with fibroids and the issue of blood is different for every woman but the shame and the pain is familiar to many women. My disclaimer is; what works for one person may or may not work for the next person. With that being said I am going to be as open and transparent as I possibly can when talking about my experience. I have read many blogs and post where women secretly discuss their issues while looking for some type of cure or relief. In my research in seeking for answers to my own shameful questions; I have discovered that women hide behind computer screens and blogs to ask the shameful questions that no one is willing to openly discuss. As I share my experience of living with fibroids and the issue of blood I write from a place of being naked and unashamed. In return my hopes and desires are that women who are living with fibroids or the issue of blood are set free from the shame and humiliation of fibroids or the issue of blood. This book was birth out of the pain of one woman living with fibroids and the issue of blood. However, there are thousands of women who suffer from the pain within. In life we go through things that can sometimes leave you angry and bitter. I didn't want fibroids or the issue of blood to cripple my mind or heart to hate life. I endured the pain and suffering and in return I found strength and a stronger women who lived in me. My prayers are that this book encourages women, young and old and it brings healing to your mind, body, spirit and soul. I pray that you have peace to comfort you in the midst of your pain. I pray that every woman who suffers from fibroids or the issue of blood be made whole.

Isolation

Fibroids can cause a woman to be bed ridden depending on the size, location, and the type of fibroids that a woman has. From the age of 38 to 43, I suffered with fibroids and heavy bleeding. I often experienced embarrassing and shameful moments. I stayed on my menstrual cycle for 7 days and there were times where I would come on twice a month. My fibroids were so bad; I had blood clots falling out of me that ranged from the size of a golf ball to the size of a grapefruit. I bled from February 2013 until September 2013 everyday none stop. I messed up clothes, sheets, car seats and anything else that I sat down on. Oftentimes when I would take a bath, the tub would be full of blood. I would get out the tub to run some clean water in the process of running more water; I would bleed all over the bathroom floor. Towels were my best friend. I always had to have towels handy because I never knew when I was going to have an embarrassing moment. I went through so many depends, pads and tampons it was unreal and scary. I bled so much I thought I was going to bleed to death.

I remember going to a job interview and as the interview was coming to an end, I felt this really warm feeling and blood began to gush out of me as I was sitting in my chair. I knew I had to leave or it wasn't going to be good. I was glad that the interview was over but I had one problem. I had a clot that was trying to escape from my pads and I needed to leave the interview immediately. As I was leaving out the door a blood clot rolled down my pants leg and fell onto the ground. I kicked it alongside the sidewalk and walked to my car crying. My pants were soiled with blood and my self-esteem was shot to pieces. I left the interview feeling ashamed and embarrassed. I left hoping that no one saw what had happened. I got to my car and put three towels in my seat and proceeded to drive home. When I got home I put my clothes in the washer machine and got in the tub.

Another time I was at the license branch and I felt my bottom getting really warm; I guess you can say that was my sign that it wasn't going to be good for me. I got up from the chair that I was sitting in only to discover that I had blood in the chair. I left in tears because I was embarrassed. I drove home and did the same routine as I always did, I took a bath and washed my clothes and got in the bed. Black pants were my best friend even though it didn't matter what color I had on because all moments were embarrassing.

I remember when I was living in Baltimore I was feeling alone and isolated. I thought if I went to visit my two sons I would feel better. I brought a train ticket and off I went to Chicago. On the second day of my stay I was home with my youngest son John. I remember saying to him; John, I am about to take a bath listen out for me because I don't feel well; "He said ok momma" but, why are you going to take a bath and you don't feel well; I said because I am a mess and I need to go clean myself up. "He said ok, I understand" I will listen out for you. Ten minutes into my bath I began to feel dizzy. I got out of the tub to use the toilet and I began to feel really hot and my ears started popping; I eased my body to the bathroom floor where it was cooler with hopes my body temperature would cool down without me passing out. As I laid on the bathroom floor I felt really weak. I finally mustard up enough strength to call John to come help me; but he couldn't hear me. As I was going in and out of consciousness and my eyesight was blurred; John eventually came into the bathroom but when he opened the bathroom door you could tell that he was shocked to see so much blood everywhere.

There was blood in the tub and on the bathroom floor and all over the toilet. I asked John to get some extra towels and wet them in cold water then place the towels on my head, neck, face and chest until I told him to stop. I explained to him how the cold towels would help to bring my body temperature down. I then said to him if I pass out call the paramedics and then call your brother Paris. I told him not to freak out or get all weird on me because I needed him to pay attention to what I was saying to him. When I came around to myself and my ears stop ringing and my body temperature had calmed down to a calming state; I then said to John call the paramedics and then call your brother. When the paramedics arrived they said "It looks like a crime scene in here let's get her out of here she is losing too much blood". I glanced over at John and he was looking at me with fear in his eyes as though he was about to lose his mother. When we got down stairs the paramedics proceeded to put me inside the ambulance. Paris arrived and told John to get in the car with him and they followed the ambulance as they rushed me to the hospital. When the doctor came to see me I was told my hemoglobin was really low and I needed a blood transfusion and I should consider having a hysterectomy. I was given IV fluids for dehydration and later released and told to follow up with my primary care doctor.

The next day I went to do some work at the business center located in the condominium high rise where Paris lived. I figured if I did some work it would help me to get my mind off my issue; little did I know; I was about to face another embarrassing moment. I felt that warm feeling again, sure enough when I got up; I had blood in the chair that I was sitting in. I cleaned the chair up and began to walk to the elevator back to my sons unit when blood clots began to fall down my legs. As I walked to the elevator I began to cry. I was so embarrassed because there were other people who were in the business center who saw me in my shameful moment. One of the managers came up to me and asked me was everything ok; then she said is there anything that I can do to help you? With tears in my eyes I said yes; could you please help me back to my sons unit? I really didn't want her help but I was so embarrassed to walk alone I accepted her help. After I told her that I had fibroids and that was the reason I was bleeding so badly she showed great compassion for me and told me to call her if I needed anything. Once I arrived to my sons unit I got in the tub and soaked myself in a puddle of tears. I sat there wishing, hoping and praying that one day the pain, suffering and bleeding would stop.

Blood can cause a person to be isolated because of the smell of blood. After bleeding so much and for such a long period of time the color of my blood had changed to three different shades of red. There were times my blood was bright red, then it would be dark red, then it would change to a really dark red almost like a burgundy color. I noticed that my blood would sometimes have a smell to it. There were other women in whom I communicated with on different blog sites who had some of the same experiences as I did suggested that I could have been possibly experiencing signs of my fibroids dying off. How true that was I can't say but it did bring hope to me in my time of need if that was really happening. When I told the doctor what I was experiencing he felt that it was a possibility that I was shedding old blood; he didn't know for certain but that was the answer he gave to me in theory.

Nevertheless, because of the constant bleeding and wearing pads all day my butt checks developed blisters. My skin begin to break down because it wasn't able to breathe from the daily buildup of moisture. The moisture also caused the lips of my vagina to blister. There were times where I had to relieve myself from all the pads by putting a lot of towels under me for about an hour or two so that I could allow my butt and vagina to breathe. This was unsanitary but when you are trying to find some form of relief you will try anything.

At this particular time of my life I was married and facing a harsh reality of a divorce. The constant pain and heavy bleeding left me unable to make love to my husband. I would oftentimes stay locked up in our bedroom not wanting to be bothered with my husband because of the constant pain that I was in. There were also times where the pain was so great I didn't want to eat. There were other times where I would pray that my husband wouldn't smell me. I stayed cleaning myself up but it was still embarrassing at times when I didn't smell like a fresh bed of roses. There would be times where I would lay in bed and silently cry wishing that I was dead. I got tired of going to the doctor only to here that my hemoglobin was 5.0 and I needed blood. I also got tired of doctors wanting to give me a blood transfusion which I never accepted. I felt like I was an alien from another planet.

At that time of my life I was done having children but I didn't want a hysterectomy. There were other options that were given to me but none of them was any better than the other. The list of options that I was given was uterine embolization which is done by burning the lining of a woman's uterus. Birth control pills which I took but they didn't work for me; the Depo-Provera shot which I took in a form of one shot which escalated my bleeding. Another option was to have an IUD which is a T-shape flexible device inserted into my uterus which I didn't do. The other option was a Myomectomy which is done by removing the fibroids; I was also offered to have a D&C which is a brief surgical procedure in which the cervix is dilated and a special instrument is used to scrape the uterine lining. The last option was a hysterectomy. After hearing my options I felt depressed and hopeless. Once I done some research, I realized that the options that were given to me wasn't any better than my current situation; in fact those options that was given to me had the potential to result in possible side effects that could be worse than the current issue that I was dealing with.

When the pain was really unbearable I wore my pain on my face. Dealing with the issue of blood and fibroids would oftentimes leave me feeling emotionally drained. I had moments where I believed that the bleeding would stop and the fibroids would shrink; but there were also times when I would say "Why me, please Lord take me or the blood away."

One of the many things that I have learned while living with fibroids and the issue of blood is; you will oftentimes find yourself feeling angry, sad, depressed, bitter, and frustrated. Living with the issue of blood and having fibroids can also make you feel as though you are being tormented in your mind. When agony shows up the struggle becomes that much worst. I often felt like I was wearing a wet diaper that was always in need of changing. I found myself in constant pain because I couldn't take the pain of having fibroids and my monthly cramps at the same time. There were so many times where I had to call off work because I couldn't leave the house without bleeding through my clothes. There were times where I would have to leave work because I had bled through my clothes. I felt alone and discouraged when I couldn't leave my home or when I couldn't talk to anyone about all that I was going through. I felt like a prisoner in my own mind and body.

Although, I have a relationship with the Lord and faith that can move mountains; I sometimes thought that Jesus wasn't hearing my cries. When sickness shows up it is truly a testing of your faith. If you were to ask me my definition of sickness, I would say sickness creeps into your body and leaves no remorse as to how and what it does to a person mentally or physically. In my experience sickness will test what you believe.

In the midst of it all I learned how to find strength in my weakness. Living with the issue of blood and fibroids placed a new demand on my life. It forced me to find a new level of endurance that I didn't know I had. I am grateful for the finding because it really caused for me to stretch into parts of me that I didn't know existed. I would like to encourage you to not give up even when the pain becomes unbearable. My prayers are that you don't allow isolation to take over, and that you fight with all that is inside of you. My prayers are that you dig deeper until you reach another level of strength and endurance. Be encouraged.

Shame

I remember buying panties and throwing them away as though they were a piece of tissue. One of my most embarrassing moments was when I had to wear depends. I remember one day I was at the unemployment office and somehow the topic of fibroids came up between me and another lady and this was her exact words to me. She stated, "I almost lost my mind when I had fibroids". She also said, "I had to take an anti-depressant because I was ready to commit suicide." "She said that she wouldn't wish for her worst enemy to have fibroids". I looked at her with tears in my eyes because I knew the pain in which she was describing. I secretly felt the same as she did. There were times where I couldn't bring myself to pray because of all the frustration and pain that I was in. When moments like that would occur I would lie in bed and ask the Lord to keep my mind. When I couldn't utter a word with tears running down my face I would confess in my mind saying; Lord please, please, please, keep my mind in all of this. I remember going through the process of having really bad out breaks where my face was full of bumps and brown spots, my hair had fallen out and I had excessive weight gain. I experienced pain in my joints and I was always fatigued. I continually lived in fear as to when my next embarrassing moment was going to be.

After experiencing so many shameful moments I no longer wanted to be out amongst people but I knew I couldn't live my life locked away. I felt discouraged and disappointed because I had very little support or encouragement in my time of need. I couldn't believe there were so many women living with fibroids that were not willing to share their experience to help or encourage other women. I realize that some things are personal but what I don't understand is; when the topic of fibroids is brought up; why do women shut down and act as though if you talk about fibroids you are telling a dirty little secret that isn't supposed to be discussed. Sometimes when I would share my embarrassing moments with other women they would look at me with a facial expression that screamed "Better you then me." While other women would voice their thoughts of how they couldn't bear what I was going through, or they would say things like "I hope you find a solution to your problem good luck." I would be so angry I told myself that I would never share my experience with anyone else because the shame was so great.

After all the nasty and rude comments or gestures that some women would say or make I couldn't believe they would have the nerve to say, "I will be praying for you." My thoughts were thanks but no thanks. Once I began to get negative feedback I stop discussing my experience in great details. I began to only share small pieces about my experience but nothing to graphic. I came to the realization that no one wanted to share their shameful moments. I would have days where I felt like I was on an emotional roller coaster because I couldn't understand how fibroids or the issue of blood could have such power over someone and impact a person's life in such a debilitating way. I also couldn't understand how living with fibroids or the issue of blood could change my life in such a shameful and humiliating way. I was baffled at the thought of knowing that I had something that was growing inside of me and it wasn't a baby.

I must admit out of all my shameful moments that I have ever experienced in life this thing called fibroids and the issue of blood had to be the worst by far. I didn't realize blood could take so much away from you that it could immobilize you when lost rapidly. The shame of living with the issue of blood and fibroids had taken up residency in my mind and in my heart. When you are plagued with a sickness you will learn that it takes precedence over everything in your life. Shame was the driver but blood and fibroids was the root when the three get together that is a formula for disaster. Another thing that I have learned in this experience as it pertains to shame is; the end of a thing is better than the beginning and you have to believe that at some point there will be light at the end of the tunnel but you will have to press and fight to see the end. Darkness can and will overtake you when you walk in agreement with it; shame can cause you to be mute, or wish that you wasn't alive to feel the pain.

Imagine having a question that you want to ask but you know it would sound so far-fetched to the virgin ear that hasn't experienced pain in the magnitude in which you have; so you keep the questions to yourself with hopes that one day you would be able to ask someone so that you can get an answer to your problem. You secretly hope that one day you can speak about your experience without someone judging you. You secretly hope that one day someone will talk about the ugly and shameful experiences of living with fibroids or the issue of blood.

Shame invites itself in, in so many ways. One of my many shames that I carried in the back of my mind while living with fibroids and the issue of blood was; if I shared my true story with another woman would she judge me if my condition was worst then hers?

Whenever I would talk about fibroids with other women my hopes were that she would share her experience and maybe we could find some type of cure or remedy together but that never happened. Most women become tolerant of living with fibroids or the issue of blood until they absolutely can't bear the pain anymore, at least that was my case. Also, another shameful fact is many women don't have health insurance to obtain the care that is needed. My prayers are that you are freed from shame. My hopes are to put faces to the many women who are suffering with fibroids or the issue of blood. My prayers are that you be encouraged and that you expose light to the dark places that has caused you to live in shame. My prayers are that you no longer be bound by shame. Be encouraged.

Helpless

I can recall so many times I felt helpless and afraid. I felt like the doctors were not hearing my concerns. I remember I went to one doctor and he examined me and after he was done examining me he said to me; my suggestion to you would be that you consider having a hysterectomy. I already knew what my options were as far as having a surgical procedure done. I was hoping there was some type of medication that I could have taken to stop the bleeding. I was hurt and angry when the doctor first suggestion was to have a hysterectomy. I looked at the doctor with tears rolling down my face and I said to him "If I was your mother, daughter, wife, sister, or granddaughter would that be the first option that you would give to them? He looked at me and said nothing. I put my clothes on and walked out of his office.

I remember feeling empty and helpless. After leaving the doctor's office I felt like I was some type of experimental animal that no one had a cure for. It seemed as though every time that I went to the doctor which was often I left feeling worst then when I went in. Whatever piece of hope that I held onto in order to live or survive this life of torment and despair; each doctor that I went to, ripped me apart piece by piece with their negative words. I had moments where I lost hope of ever seeing myself healed. I felt as though I was given a death sentence and all options pointed to the road of helplessness.

Once I started doing more research I found out there were women from all over the world who was dealing with the same issue. We were all seeking a solution on how to stop the heavy bleeding or how to shrink or get rid of fibroids. Some of the women who I had spoken with stated "when they stopped eating meat they didn't bleed so heavily while other women stated their fibroids stopped growing completely. I didn't know how true that was but I figured; what did I have to lose, so I stop eating meat. As I continued to research I found out that certain foods and meats have hormones in them which can cause the fibroids to grow larger in size. Equipped with my new information I changed my eating habits and I started taking organic apple cider vinegar and baking soda along with blackstrap molasses and my bleeding stopped. It finally stopped after a daunting 7 months and returned back to a regular once a month painful menstrual cycle. Another thing that I did was I cut out sugars and breads or foods that carried high levels of yeast. I was on a strict eating regiment which worked for me as far as my everyday bleeding was concerned. I still was in pain from the fibroids and I still had the heavy bleeding when I came on my menstrual cycle; however, I was glad about one thing; I wasn't bleeding every day.

When I was researching information and possible solutions or a cure that would get rid of fibroids there was so much stuff on the internet it made me feel even more helpless. I felt like everyone had tapped into a get rich quick scheme for curing fibroids. There are so many so called quick fixes or solutions for getting rid of fibroids on the internet, if you are not careful, you can make things worse for yourself. This is why I gave the disclaimer; what works for someone else may or may not work for you. Whenever I came across a piece of information it always gave me hope that maybe I found something that would work for me and my condition. Then I would lose all hope after trying it and finding out that it didn't work for me.

Talk about feeling helpless and hopeless; yelp that was me. I would be so disappointed when I came across information where people were charging such ridiculous prices for a cure for fibroids that they claimed to work only to discover that the products lack effectiveness of curing fibroids. I am not going to even talk about all the time, money, energy and effort I spent on searching for a cure or relief for fibroids and the issue of blood. I will say this; my time and efforts were endless. I was always hoping to find something that would give me some type of relief or cure; I didn't consider my efforts or time to be in vain. However, the products that I did find only gave short term relief if any. The organic apple cider vinegar worked for a little while but it didn't get rid of my fibroids.

My inner strength wouldn't allow me to give up totally although there were so many days that I wanted to. My two sons kept encouraging me while I was enduring this new life of horror. Even-though they didn't fully understand all that I was going through they were able to see how much distress I was in. I never stopped fighting because there is a fighter that lives within me. However, I did have a lot of moments where my faith and strength was put on trial. My sons would say to me, "It's going to be alright you will find something or we will find something." They would also say, "Keep doing what you are doing until something better comes along that will work for you." Paris and John brought so much hope to me when I needed it the most. They loved me in spite of my many mood swings and through my tears and my embarrassing moments, and for that, I will always be grateful.

When you are in a hopeless situation it isn't always easy to speak with hope or see hope when your situation says something differently. Most of the time you can't see the end when everything appears to be dark and the end that you do see doesn't have a great outcome. Oftentimes then not when you are going through something you will speak from the place that is causing you the greatest pain. Your words are often driven from a place of pain, shame and frustration. No one wants to go through something and not have someone by their side, someone who is driven to encourage you when you can't encourage yourself. Someone to advocate for you when you can't advocate for yourself; when you have a need you expect to have someone to carry the burden with you and take the time to learn what you are going through; so when it seems as though you are losing hope, you will have someone who is still fighting for you who knows the process in which you are in.

Be encouraged as you travel through this process rather it be alone or with someone and remember that you are not alone and one day this too shall pass. Don't give up;

fight until you get the expected end of what you desire for your health. Don't stop fighting until you are healed or until you get the relief that you desire. My prayers are that you keep your body as healthy as possible. Don't give up because together we can fight the ugly war against fibroids and the issue of blood. I would always tell myself that giving up wasn't an option; if I gave up, I would fail myself. I would tell myself that my life is worth living and I have victory even if my situation appears to show me something different. I always knew deep down inside that I wasn't going to always live a life that was filled with so much pain and suffering as it pertained to my physical health. I would also say things like I have greatness inside of me. I will not die with this issue and I will fight even in my weakness. I will fight in my brokenness with hopes that one day I will be made whole. I knew that I was born a fighter so deep down in my soul I knew I couldn't let fibroids take my mind or win the fight. I knew that I was an eagle and I had to soar higher then what I was going through. Did I lose hope at times? Yes, but I would pick hope back up and fight the battle that was before me until I received a healthier expected end.

Oftentimes the expected end that you look for doesn't exactly play out the way that you would foresee it to be. However, it works out being what is best for you at that time. Sometimes the things that we are against turn out to work together for our good. Everyone results will be different but the expected outcome is the same which is relief or healing. You have to do what works for you. Stay encouraged and if you have lost hope, pick hope back up and don't stop fighting until you are satisfied with your expected end. Remember that the choices and decisions in which you will have to make need to come from a place of peace. The end result should be that you are healthy and that you can live life being the best person that you were created to be. My prayers are that you no longer live in a place of helplessness and you see yourself healed. My prayers are that if you are walking this fibroids journey alone that you join with other women and stand together. Be encouraged.

Lord Please Keep My Mind Through It All

There were so many times were I felt lost, abandoned, frustrated, weary and paralyzed. I felt like I had no support or comfort in the midst of my storm. I would sometimes lie awake in great pain uttering the words; "Lord Please Keep my mind Through it All" because there were moments when I felt like I was slipping away into a dark place called depression. I would pray healing scriptures over myself; I would lay heads on myself; and confess healing over my mind, body, spirit and soul. It seemed like nothing was changing, it seemed as though things got worse before they got better.

I would watch spiritual teachings, I read books, I read my bible, I listened to other women on YouTube talk about snippets of their experience while living with fibroids or the issue of blood, and I did meditation. I tried just about everything to keep my mind built up so that I wouldn't fall weak to all that I was going through. I wanted to try something natural to shrink the fibroids or to stop the heavy flow of my bleeding; so I went to see a doctor who specialized in herbs and natural healing. I was given a tea that was made from many different herbs. I was instructed to take the tea once a month when I came on my menstrual cycle. The tea that I was given was awful and unfortunately it didn't help. I often thought about the woman in the bible who dealt with the issue of blood. I found myself being able to identify with her embarrassing and hopeless moments. I felt like an outcast. It is a horrible feeling when you feel displaced and you feel as though you don't fit anywhere. Seclusion can make you feel like you don't exist. I would pray daily for some type of cure for fibroids so that I wouldn't have to send my body through so many harsh surgeries. I prayed daily that my womb would get better and the bleeding would subside to a normal state.

I was always hoping that one day a woman who had experienced the pain and suffering of living with fibroids and the issue of blood would talk about her most shameful and embarrassing moments in details. I was looking for a woman to speak about how she coped with fibroids or what she found to work for her, if anything. I wanted her to talk about the pain in which she suffered and her embarrassing moments of living with fibroids or the issue of blood. I wasn't looking for any woman to speak about fibroids. I was looking for a woman who had been shamed enough by her painful experiences of living with fibroids or the issue of blood. I wasn't looking for a woman who had minimal experience, minimal pain, or minimal shame. I was waiting to hear from a woman who was bold enough to talk about her true experiences without holding back what her truth was while living with fibroids. I was looking for a woman whose heart had been scarred enough by the shame of it all to share her experience of living with fibroids or the issue of blood. I wanted her to share her journey with other women so that I didn't feel like I was alone. I wasn't looking for her to talk about what she thought or felt about fibroids or the issue of blood. I wanted her to share her true cost, experience, shame, suffering and her pain of living with fibroids or the issue of blood. When I began to write this book I realized that the woman that I was looking for was me.

As I stated before not all women will experience the same type of pain because fibroids will effect every woman differently. This is why I wanted to hear from a woman or women whose experiences were harsh or brutal. I would often hear or read about what statistics had to say, what doctors had to say, and what people who had no clue about living with fibroids or the issue of blood had to say. I must say it was all alarming to hear. What was most alarming to hear was when a male doctor would talk about women living with fibroids. I couldn't understand how some male doctors; not all, could speak about fibroids but had little understanding of a woman's true experience, pain or suffering as it pertains to a woman living with fibroids or the issue of blood. Another thing that was alarming and disappointing to me was to see how insensitive some women doctors were. I couldn't believe that some of the women doctors that I came in contact with were just as uncaring as some of the male doctors. In my experience some of the women doctors that I had seen would say things like; "if you are not looking to have any more kids why would you not consider getting a hysterectomy." Another female doctor said to me "if having more children is not the issue I don't understand why you won't consider having a hysterectomy." What both women didn't understand was it didn't matter if I wanted to have more children or not; the whole point was, I wanted to keep all of my womanly parts that I came into this world with.

I also found it to be quite alarming when others would speak about a woman who suffers from fibroids and they had absolutely no knowledge of her experience or the journey of a woman who suffers with fibroids and all that she has to endure. That tells me how much people perish from a lack of knowledge. I didn't understand how someone could speak about something that they had no understanding or knowledge of. When I would pray for my own healing; I also prayed that the Lord would help His people to understand the pain of others. One of the many lessons that I have learned in life is; it is easy for some people to speak or comment on something that they have no insight or knowledge about until the pain or suffering or sickness arrives at their front door. I believe we live in a world where people feel as though they have the right to judge another individual process or their pain. I believe people have become insensitive to others pain. I also believe people have become so judgmental and critical to the point they no longer have eyes to see that we are all human and no one wants to be sick or in pain.

Honestly speaking doctors don't know where fibroids come from. They have assumed many potential causes and developed their own theories about where fibroids come from but none are factual as to where fibroids come from or how women really get fibroids. My prayers are that better research will be done to find out where fibroids come from and how fibroids can be cured. I pray for the study of fibroids where doctors and scientist come up with a cure that isn't harsh and painful for women to endure.

I pray that women won't have to continue to undergo further damages to their bodies, womb or any other bodily parts that surrounds her womb. My prayers are that women are viewed with greater value. My prayers are that women see themselves as a Queen even when she doesn't look or feel like a queen. My prayers are that all women perform at an opulent level in life where she is wealthy in her mind, body spirit and soul. Shame comes when you allow it to hide inside of you and when you don't confront it or expose it. Ask yourself this question; why would you allow yourself to be ashamed of something that you have chosen to keep a secret?

Don't allow fibroids or the ugly experience of living with fibroids or the issue of blood keep you in bondage. Remember that you are not along and as we stand together and our voices are heard as one; one day this ugly thing called fibroids will no longer live inside the many women who suffer in silence. One day there will be a cure and a healthier way to heal fibroids. See yourself healed and believe that it won't be long before you walk in your healing. Believe that it won't be long before relief shows up for the issues in which you are experiencing. Look beyond what appears to be impossible and grab a hold to what you wish for. For those of you who don't believe in Jehovah then speak and confess positive words over yourself and into your atmosphere.

Emotions

During the course of my journey of living with fibroids and the issue of blood I found myself being in and out of my emotions. One minute I was blissful, then I was sad, then I would have moments where I would cry, then there were times I felt depressed, angry, upset and displeased. Then I had times where I felt thankful, cheerful, and balanced. As you can see I was an emotional mess. I would sometimes say to myself, I was a train wreck waiting to happen. My emotions were unhealthy and displaced. Honestly speaking, I wasn't always on point in my decision making; pending the day and the level of pain that I was experiencing, I sometimes made some bad choices. I am thankful today that I didn't make such a mess of my life but I have to admit there were some choices I could've made differently for the betterment of myself. Nevertheless, I won't fuss about it, because I can't take anything back that I have done or that I have gone through, so I will use the lessons that I have learned as a reference point of the hurdles that I have climbed.

While I was in my pain and suffering, I learned a lot about my body, myself and my health. I grew and developed a stronger sense of self-worth and confidence in spite of all that I was going through. All was not lost when it came to the final outcome of my healing. I believe that my pain, tears and suffering allowed me to see how much greater my inner strength was and how deeply rooted I was to overcome whatever challenges, obstacles or barriers that I may face. It was through my suffering that I also learned how deep my capacity was to withstand under pressure and trying times. I found a new level of endurance that broke me and then restored me. I learned that sometimes when a person goes through something perseverance is better than settling. I also learned that displaced emotions can cause you to wear your emotions on your face and react to situations by how you feel verses what is true. As I look back over some of the choices that I made out of my emotions I realized that I made a few costly mistakes but the point of it all is we live, learn and grow. I have yet to experience a lesson that I wasn't able to grow from rather it was good, bad or painful.

Your perception about how you view something will oftentimes determine your truth or reality. When I would watch women on YouTube talk about the various sizes of their fibroids or their surgical procedure I was shocked to find out how many women spoke out about having complications after their procedure. I also couldn't believe how many women were still having issues with fibroids after they had gone through menopause. I began to take a new approach so that I could experience healing through others. I looked beyond my own pain and I started helping others. When I shifted my focus it allowed me to keep my mind off of what I was going through and it gave me the strength that I needed to fight my own battle. I remember having two hour conversations empowering other women to be strong while I was fighting my own battle to live.

Sometimes I would be amazed at the strength that I had; then there were times where I found myself troubled and fighting to hold on to hope. Because I secretly battled the emotional suffering and pain of living with fibroids along with the issue of blood; I didn't disclose all that I was going through in depth with family and friends. This will also be their first time hearing about my pain and suffering. I know that many of you may be thinking, I don't think I could have exposed my dark moments about my life to the world. That was my first thought as well; but then I thought, if I want to make a difference then I have to share my pain so that others can learn about some of the discomforts that a woman can experience while living with fibroids or the issue of blood.

Women are known to be nurturers; however, many women fall short when they are in need of compassion and support to be reciprocated back to them. Oftentimes than not, most women provide care and contributes to the growth and development for others to grow and flourish while they suffer silently. I didn't realize how emotionally depleted, detached and deficient I was until I went into my reserve bank only to find out that I didn't have anything left to balance me in my time of need. I realized I didn't have anyone to speak life back into me as I did for so many others. I also realized how alone and scared I was. I was being asked to make major decisions that I was scared to make on my own. I sometimes felt that I wasn't in my right state of mind to make certain decisions because of the pain and agony I was in. I was crippled by fear and doubt and I felt like I had no one to guide me through my process besides Paris and John.

The pressure of it all made the battle that much worse. I had so many decisions to make on top of facing multiple challenges. There were days where I didn't know if I was coming or going. There were other times I couldn't stop crying and feeling sorry for myself, which left me wondering was the pain and suffering ever going to stop. Everyone has their own secret battles. Fighting fibroids and the issue of blood was one of my biggest battles that almost took my mind; this battle made me fight when I had nothing to fight with. I was fighting daily to live and to be my best person but the fibroids that resided inside of me also fought daily to live.

During this period of my life I lived a life of brokenness, low iron and barely enough energy to make it through the day. I had moments where I couldn't walk up a flight of stairs without being out of breathe. One of my everyday struggles was learning to preserve my energy to make it through the day without passing out. I found that to be a task all by itself. I learned to pull on more of my mental abilities then my physical abilities. Sometimes when I would be at work I would go into the bathroom and cry. My energy level would be so low I literally struggled to stay awake. I remember being at my desk talking to clients and taking an occasional nod while they were talking to me. It was so embarrassing. I couldn't believe that I was battling with myself to stay awake. Sometimes I would be driving and I found myself nodding at the light. I had no control over my eyes they would just close and cars would began honking at me to drive.

I oftentimes found myself crying while I was driving because I didn't like the way that I was feeling and I always feared that I would have an accident because I had no control over my lack of energy. I fought daily to be happy but there were many days where the pain won. I learned to walk in humility so that I wouldn't speak from a place of pain or hurt; but I sometimes found myself so angry because I couldn't understand why I was living in constant pain. There were times when people would say to me what is wrong with you, you are not yourself. They knew that I was in pain and on those days I didn't even try to hide the pain because those were the days that my pain level was really intolerable. My prayers are that you be encouraged and that you practice daily in keeping your mind and emotions in a place that is safe. Keep your heart guarded and your emotions balanced; remember greater is in you even when you don't feel great. My prayers are that you see yourself bigger than fibroids and the issue of blood.

Help I am Anemic

My definition of being anemic is lacking in substance or being meaningful, useful or balanced. That is how my body felt daily. Living with fibroids and the issue of blood prevented my body from functioning at the maximum level in which it was created to function. I battled with having low iron which caused my energy level to be extremely low. I would oftentimes feel fatigue and exhausted. I always knew how important blood was to the human body but I never knew that there would come a day where I would have to monitor my blood on a quarterly bases.

People who are anemic battle with finding the right kinds of foods or supplements to build their blood and iron levels. If you are anemic then you know exactly what I am talking about. Most doctors will prescribe iron pills to a person who is anemic. However, some people have been known to buy an over the counter iron pill to take which can sometimes be dangerous if you are not seeing a doctor to help monitor and prescribe the right amount of iron that your body needs. Iron pills come in many different doses and can be deadly if a person over medicates. A person who is anemic should get their blood and iron levels tested regularly to make sure that they are putting the right amount of iron into their bodies. This is important so that you won't experience an iron overload. Also, certain iron pills are harsh on the stomach and has the potential to cause constipation. I wasn't able to take the iron pills that my doctor prescribed because they were harsh on my stomach and they kept me constipated. I wanted to take something that had fewer chemicals if any at all so I took an iron pill that was made from organic vegetables and organic based products. I will share a couple of things that I found to be helpful in building my blood and iron levels up. The process that I used was a slow process but it worked for me without me having to buy stool softeners or deal with stomach aches or other harsh symptoms that come along with taking iron pills.

I used organic blackstrap molasses unsulphured; I took one teaspoon in the morning and one at night. I took Vitamin Code (healthy blood) two tablets every morning. I would sometimes blend beets and make a beet juice or I would boil the beets and eat them plain. I brought the organic beets in a can but you can buy raw beets or whatever works for you. Be careful when blending the beets and drinking too much beet juice because when you go to the bathroom you may experience your stool being red; do your research and consult with a doctor. If I made beet juice I drank one glass in the morning and one in the evening. Sometimes I would drink only one glass a day. I didn't do the beet juice too much. Again what worked for me may or may not work for you. I am just sharing a few things that I took that helped to build my blood and raised my iron levels. Some women may need more than this. I know women who have to take B-12 shoots while others have to get blood transfusions. After learning the many side effects of the medication that my doctor prescribed, I came to the conclusion that it was best that I took natural or organic products.

Before I started taking the vitamin code pills my hemoglobin would range from 5.1 to 6.0. After I started taking the vitamin code for healthy blood and incorporated eating leafy green vegetables into my diet on a daily bases my hemoglobin went up to 8.5 which was great for me especially since I was always around 5 or 6. I had one doctor to tell me that she didn't know how I was standing before her because technically I should have been getting a blood transfusion or dead, that's how frank she was with me. "She said the only answer that I can come up with to justify this is that your body has been functioning at this level for so long that it has become accustom to functioning at such a low level." "She said I have seen patients who are where you are in their hemoglobin count but they were in the hospital getting a blood transfusion." I hate to admit that the doctor was right about one thing; my body had functioned so long at a low and unbalanced state to the degree were that was my normal.

My issue of blood started from the first day of my menstrual cycle. I always had really bad and heavy menstrual cycles; but it wasn't until I turned 37 years old I started my journey with fibroids. I learned to live and cope with the deficiencies. I became numb to the pain, it was through the numbness I learned to press through the difficult times along with building a high tolerance for pain. I built up many walls and I wore many faces to hide all the pain and issues that I was dealing with while living with fibroids and the issue of blood.

I am not suggesting that you share in the negative coping skills that I had formed. I am simply sharing my experience about some of the many ways in which I coped with fibroids and the issue of blood. Because I was dealing with two different issues which was the issue of blood and fibroids my level of pain was increased deeply. Being anemic left me always feeling cold and my hands and feet would feel like I was in a deep freezer. I always had to wear layers of clothes. I slept under a blanket most of the time rather it was hot or cold. I required the heat to be on as often as I could get away with it; pending my kids didn't turn the heat off. Rather I was at work, or at home I drove people crazy with my need for heat.

Many people don't understand the affliction of being anemic or the constant and abnormal feeling of being cold. I would get remarks from people saying things like "what is wrong with you; you feel like you are dead." "You need to take something for that, you really need some help because I never seen or met anyone like you who stay cold all the time." Different places where I worked there were times when my co-workers would intentionally turn the heat off or turn the air up really high to see me be discomforted in my suffering. When I would ask why they turned the heat off or the air up there response would be, don't you have a heater. I would be so cold to the point my nose would be running. I couldn't believe how cruel and uncaring people could be.

I realized when people don't understand your pain or the distress in which you suffer compassion and mercy goes out the window. It was during those times that I prayed like never before for my strength, blood and iron levels to be restored to a normal state. I was tired of feeling ashamed for what I was going through. My current hemoglobin count is 13.0. I will explain in another chapter how I reached the point where I am today. This has been a long uphill battle as to where I was and where I am now. I would like to encourage you to keep hoping for the best because you too will walk in your healing. Believe that you are on the road of recovery and your fibroid days will be behind you soon. Believe that one day you will no longer walk in shame or pain, but you will encourage another woman as she walks and waits for her healing.

My prayers are as you continue to read each chapter I pray that it brings healing and comfort to you in your time of need. My prayers are as you continue to walk out your journey that you do it knowing that one day the issues that you are dealing with as it pertains to fibroids or the issue of blood will no longer be. Be strong and believe that you can do all things through Christ who strengthens you. I asked that you shift your mind and put it in a direction that will give you proven results and allow your thoughts to rest in a place of peace. Keep love in your heart in the midst of adversity.

No Health Insurance

Health insurance is one of the leading factors as to why many women are not able to get the quality of care that is needed when it comes to choosing the best surgical procedure that would work for them. I have talked to countless women who have said if they had health insurance they would be able to get a surgical procedure that would be suitable for them. Other women have disclosed having Medicaid but they are unable to find a quality doctor to perform the procedure that is needed. Medicaid requires many forms to be filled out and the process is time consuming to get an approval to have a hysterectomy. Also, pending what state you live in will determine your process, approval and cost. There are other concerns that women face when it comes to insurance which are; finding and maintaining affordable health insurance and finding a doctor that is in her insurance network of providers. There are also co-payments and insurance deductibles that will have to be met. If a woman has private insurance or Medicaid she will still have to get a preauthorization in order for the insurance company to pay for her procedure.

There are many stressors involved rather a woman has insurance or not. For starters she has to choose what surgical procedure she feels would work best for her along with finding a doctor who has experience in doing surgical procedures pertaining to fibroids or a doctor who is experienced in performing hysterectomies. She also has to go through a series of test and exams to see if she is healthy enough to have the surgical procedure done that her and her doctor have agreed upon. Some of the concerns that women have are; who will help them while they are recovering? Also, if she works another concern will be does she have enough time up at work to take off to allow the proper healing for her body? Also, does she have enough money to cover her bills while she is out of work?

If a woman doesn't have private insurance and she has Medicaid she has to find a good doctor who accepts Medicaid and who has the surgical experience in removing fibroids or performing hysterectomies. A woman who has Medicaid faces a greater shortage in selecting from her pool of doctors who can perform her procedure. She will find out that her options will be very slim simply because there are not many doctors who accept Medicaid that does a great job or have the experience with performing hysterectomies or the removal of fibroids. A woman who has Medicaid can sometimes face a higher risk of getting her procedure done at a replicable hospital. Another concern that she would have to take into consideration would be; if the hospital is known for having excessive mal-practice suits and does the hospital have a reputation where people walk in but they don't walk out.

These are some of the things that I faced when I went through my process rather I had private insurance or Medicaid. I am sure that these will be some of the concerns that will enter into the minds of other women as they decide on what surgical procedure will work best for them. There are many barriers that are at hand when it comes to insurance in America. I believe because of insurance barriers and the high cost of insurance many Americans have poor health, especially women. I also believe that people who don't have healthcare insurance are treated differently from people who have private insurance or Medicaid.

Doctors and hospitals will often bill a patient insurance company at the higher rate which oftentime will leave the patient to pay higher balances for their co-pays after their surgery and services have been completed. Most private insurance companies will cover you at 80% leaving the patient with a remaining balance of 20%. I was in such disbelief when I received my bills for the total cost of my surgery. My eyeballs nearly bulged out of my head when I saw that my surgery totaled almost $30,000; which was equivalent to one person's annual salary. The 20% that was left for me to pay was very high as well which lead me to apply for hardship assistance. This is why I gave the comparison of cost between someone who has private insurance and someone who has Medicaid because the difference is substantially larger for someone who has private insurance.

When I received my bills in the mail I was sadden by the high cost because I knew in my heart my procedure shouldn't have totaled the amount in which I was billed for. I was also grieved by the many high charges that I was left to pay. Some women, not all; will also face another set of concerns which are; who will care for their child or children if kids are involved; also, who is going to do the shopping, cleaning, cooking and washing, especially if she is a woman with limited resources, money, assistance or family. Women who don't have any insurance at all tend to face bigger issues opposed to women who have private insurance or a woman who has Medicaid. A woman who doesn't have any insurance or the suitable income to cover her expenses for surgery; her experience will escalate to a greater level of pain.

The reason why I say this is because she will be asked to put a large amount of money down before a doctor would even touch her. She will be asked to pay so much up front and then a portion mid-way before she have her surgery and then she will be expected to pay her balance after her surgery is completed. Rather you have insurance or not they all come with their own set of issues or barriers. There are a small percentage of people who have insurance that will cover at one hundred percent. Again, this goes back to what I stated before. Every woman situation is different; I am just one woman who has chosen to be open about sharing my experience as it pertains to insurance. What I have experienced in this process is when women are faced with a major decision to make about their well-being it can become mentally and physically draining; especially when it comes to her making the best decision about her quality of life.

Oftentimes I would question myself about my decision and the timing in which I had chosen to move forward to have my surgery. After evaluating all of my options I said to myself, Renita, there isn't going to be a so call right time to have this surgery if you are tired of being in pain and you can't take the shame and embarrassing moments any longer and you have health insurance through your job that will pay for your procedure; then why not do it now. With the help of my mother I made the choice to move forward with having my surgery. I stop thinking about everything else that would have told me that my timing was off and now wasn't a good time.

When I looked back from the time of when I first started my journey with fibroids I realized my timing was always off. I told myself that I had to make the time if I wanted to have a better quality of life. I know that this may sound silly or crazy to some; but I couldn't even allow my finances to be an issue while I was out of work or anything else. Another barrier that I was faced with was the day before my surgery I was terminated from my job. The reason that I was given by HR was; because I wasn't employed at my job for a year and I didn't have enough sick time accumulated to take off for a month and my vacation time wasn't effective until I worked a full year for the company I was told they wouldn't be able to hold my position for the time period in which I needed. I was also told if my position was still available I was more than welcome to reapply. I had only been employed with the company for seven months; their company policy stated that a worker could take six weeks of unpaid leave if it was after their ninety day grace period. However, I had already taken a leave of absence five months prior to me requesting the time off for my surgery. I was involved in a car accident which required me to be off for six weeks so that I could attend physical therapy. Talk about timing being off.

My choice still remained the same to have the surgery. I walked out of my director office and turned in all of my keys and proceeded to walk out the building. I remember saying as I walked out the building, this too shall pass. After I had my surgery and some of the pain had subsided I filed for unemployment benefits. Talk about obstacles and facing challenges. I found out a month after my claim was filed and pending review the company that I had previously worked for didn't pay into unemployment benefits. That was a blow right to my stomach which was already tender. Through all of this I didn't stop believing that things were going to work out for me. I didn't know how, but I knew that it would. My oldest son who is an entrepreneur, who always has some type of business venture going on, called me and said; I have some work that needs to be done on the computer. "He said if you are interested let me know and I will pay you. Also, let me know when you would be able to start. I said ok. As I worked from home on the things that my son needed me to do; I also worked on writing this book which was birth out of my pains and setbacks.

The other issue that I faced after I was terminated from my job was; I had 30 days from the date in which I was terminated to still be eligible for my health insurance benefits. I had a post opt appointment to attend, blood work that needed to be drawn along with a final visit to see the doctor and another eight week checkup before my insurance would end. All of my appointments ended up happening in the time frame of the 30 days in which I was still covered under my insurance except the last eight week checkup. I encouraged myself not to worry and I shifted my focus on having a healthy recovery. I also encouraged myself by reminding myself not to focus on the minor things because what was major had already been taken care of. I reminded myself to live in my today and not to worry about my tomorrows because my tomorrows held their own set of problems, troubles, worries and stressors. I would like to encourage you to stay positive and believe that provision has already been made on your behalf. I want to encourage you that whatever method that you might have to use as far as insurance goes rather it be self-pay, Medicaid, or private insurance be diligent in your research and do what works best for you. Be encouraged and know that every woman will have a different outcome and every woman will have to choose what works best for her.

Be encouraged and be the difference in which you want to see. My prayers are when you feel in doubt get in a quiet place and ask for guidance and direction. My prayers are that you hold people accountable and don't be concerned about the minor things because what is most important is how you bounce back from it all. Be encouraged and be content with whatever choice you make and don't allow anyone to take your freedom of choice away from you.

The Beast Within

It is a horrible feeling to have something living inside of you that causes you great pain. Two months prior to my scheduled surgery I went to the doctor to get my annual checkup and my doctor told me that my fibroids had gotten bigger and they were sitting in a place that could potentially cause other problems if they weren't removed. My doctor asked me to schedule a second appointment so that she could do a transvaginal ultrasound. I scheduled my appointment two weeks later and boy did I get an eye opener. While my doctor was performing the ultrasound she told me if I wanted to observe the examination I could do so by looking at the flat screen that was located on the wall. I was amazed by the new technology but that was short lived. Shortly after the doctor began to show me my many fibroids and their location I began to cry. As I was looking at the screen I saw images of a ball, then another image that looked as though I was carrying a baby. I saw another image that looked like a monster was attached to the lining of my uterus. I couldn't understand how something that looked like some type of alien was living inside of me and it wasn't a baby. My thoughts and emotions were all over the place. I felt sad, angry, confused, bitter and overwhelmed.

After viewing the images from the ultrasound I must admit they painted a horrible image in my mind and left me even the more scared. I remember saying to God; how is it that you are the giver of life; but yet I have something that is living inside of me that is trying to take my life. Something that was living inside of me that was sharing my blood supply. I couldn't understand all that was going on because each thought left my mind feeling more confused and puzzled as to what was happening to me internally. I was told that I had four fibroids inside of me that my doctor was able to see from the results of the ultrasound; but later I was told by the doctor who was actually going to perform my surgery that there could be more fibroids inside of me but he wouldn't know until he actually perform the surgery. My doctor said that sometimes fibroids hide behind other organs inside of a woman's body and not all the time will the fibroids be able to be seen when an ultrasound is done pending there location.

After I had my surgery I found that to be true because I had multiple fibroids that were located in another location where the ultrasound wasn't able to detect. After I had my ultrasound I couldn't tell anyone what I had seen because I felt so embarrassed and ashamed to even repeat what I saw or what I thought I saw. The flip side of that was even if I did mention what I saw I probably would have been viewed as crazy. Most definitely I would have been misunderstood as to what I was trying to convey about how I felt after my examination. When I would share my experience with other women they would be grossed out. However; I did come across some women who were encouraged and happy to hear that they were not the only one battling with fibroids in such a distressing way. Every now and again I would share a couple of graphic photos which resembled images of a miscarriage but that wasn't often.

I have been told by some doctors that fibroids could possibly be generational, they could possibly come from foods that women eat, they could come from certain hair products that women use, scar tissue, and the list goes on and on but there are no concrete facts as to where fibroids come from. This is why I named this chapter the beast within because no one knows where the beast comes from or why does a woman have the beast living inside of her. Fibroids have been known to cause a woman stomach to protrude; causing a woman to appear as though she is pregnant when she isn't. I oftentimes kept a bloated stomach; it was seldom that my stomach was flat. I frequently had to buy clothes that were bigger to somewhat camouflage how big my stomach was.

In my opinion one of the worst things to face in life is to have a problem that you are forced to live with that hinders you from living a healthy life. I believe that women go through so much in life and most of the time a lot is over looked when it comes to all that women have to bear. There is still an expectation for a woman to continue to perform even when she is in a weak state. It's like the first time that she shows any signs of life she is considered to be ok. When sometimes the reality is she is still in a battle but no one can see her pain because all that is known of her is the strength that she possesses. Oftentimes a true evaluation of her current condition isn't taking into consideration. Every woman is strong in her own way but even the strong falls weak at times. It's not enough to say or present yourself to be strong when you have an inner battle going on inside of you that screams that you are weak and you need help. The majority of women tend to keep doing and doing and doing without taking the necessary time that is needed to be restored from all that she gives out. Family, friends, doctors, or significant other; are not fully aware of what a woman goes through or the extent of her pain while living with fibroids or the issue of blood. My desire is to inform others about the beast that lives within with hopes that better research methods are produced from the cries and pain of women all over the world.

Many women will fight to the bitter end but at what cost and how much would it cost her. The beast that lives within can cause some women to lose heart because after you have been in a battle for so long you will eventually get tired. It's just like a professional boxer; once they go twelve rounds if they make it too twelve rounds and the referee announces the winner; one would think by looking at the fight that whoever is left standing won. Which is true in that sense; but if it was a fight that caused for them to take some punches that were unfamiliar or more painful than what they have experienced; then you won't see the bruises on the outside as much as you would the inside. What I am alluding to is some pains and bruises won't present themselves to be visible for everyone to see because the damage that has been done will be internal.

My prayers are that you don't give up and that you continue to fight. My prayers are that you won't allow others to put more on you then what you can really bear while you are in your own personal battle. My prayers are that you don't lose hope and that you stand even in your time of need. My prayers are when you feel weak that the Lord will lift your arms and place the right person, tools and resources to assist you. My prayers are that your pain and suffering will come to an end and that you live a life that is healthy and productive. My prayers are that as you deal with the issue of blood or fibroids that your end result brings forth a new beginning that will allow you a new outlook on life. My prayers are that you don't grow to be bitter in your journey. Be encouraged and make each day count towards your healing and see yourself where you want to be.

Blood

I must admit I battled with writing this chapter because I didn't want to get into a crash course about human blood; I also didn't want to gross anyone out by talking about all of my graphic moments and experiences of dealing with the issue of blood. So with that being said I will keep this chapter short and simple and only discuss a few of my experiences.

What made me decide to try the depo shot was when I went to bible study on a Thursday night after having a very shameful and humiliating experience. I was enjoying the worship experience and forty five minutes into the church service I began to feel my bottom get really warm and I knew that wasn't a good sign. As I proceeded to get up from the chair that I was sitting in which was burgundy in color, I noticed that the chair was stained with blood. I was glad that I was wearing black pants but that didn't stop how embarrassed I felt for messing up the church chair. Honestly speaking, it wasn't about the church chair. It had everything to do with the shame of the issue of blood and the fact that if I didn't leave at the time when I left, I was about to pass a clot which would have left further shame and embarrassment.

When I left the church crying that was my breaking point to try something different. I had thought about trying something new for a while however; I had never been a fan of taking medicine other than an alieve for pain when I would come on my menstrual cycle. As I researched possible methods and I spoke to other women who stated that the depo shot stop their bleeding for months or even years; I made an appointment to speak to my doctor to see how she felt about me taking the depo shot seeing how my tubes were already tied, clipped and burned. My doctor didn't see a problem with me taking the depo shot she actually welcomed the idea and told me to set up another appointment so that I could get the depo shot. My doctor wanted to put me on birth control pills but I opted out to take the depo shot.

Taking the depo shot was one of the worst mistakes that I had ever made. I had experienced an adverse reaction to the shot, instead of the depo shot helping to subside my bleeding it made me bleed profusely and longer. When I got the depo shot I didn't know that I had fibroids. After I took the depo shot and I got my first menstrual cycle I noticed that it was going on ten days and I was still bleeding, then it was fifteen days and I was still bleeding. This is when I knew something was wrong and this is when I started my seven month journey of non-stop bleeding. I always had the issue of blood but never did I go past the seven days of my monthly menstrual cycle. I went back to the doctor and my doctor tried to offer me another depo shot; I declined the shot. My words to her was "if my first reaction to taking the depo shot has caused me to bleed heavier and worst then my original state why would I want to take another shot." I wanted to allow the first shot to run out of my system. Little did I know that the depo shot was about to be one of my biggest and worst nightmares ever. When I went back to the doctor to find out why I was still bleeding the doctors couldn't understand why I had been bleeding for so long and I only had one depo shot. I had been to countless emergency rooms and none of the doctors were able to tell me why I was bleeding and clotting so heavily.

After five months of clotting and bleeding I went to see another doctor and I explained to him my many experiences of going to the ER and going to see other doctors and the outcomes of each visit. The doctor examined me and then he gave me a referral to go to a clinic where I was able to get a free vaginal ultrasound. Once my test results came back it revealed that I had fibroids. After I found out that I had fibroids one of the specialist said to me that I shouldn't have taken the depo shot because it can cause a woman who has fibroids to bleed worse. I told the doctor when I took the depo shoot I didn't know that I had fibroids.

The new doctor stated he could prescribe something to possibly stop the bleeding but the medicine would require that I have insurance, but of course, at that time I didn't have any insurance. The medicine was so expensive I couldn't afford to pay for it out of pocket. I don't remember the name of the medicine and it is probably best that I don't because I wouldn't want anyone else who doesn't have health insurance to be disappointed as I was. The doctor also stated that the insurance company has to give authorization for that particular medication. Because I didn't have any health insurance he then gave me birth control pills in hopes that my bleeding would stop. Needless to say that didn't work; he later prescribed me a different birth control pill, that didn't work either. He gave me progestogen pills and those didn't help either. I decided to stop taking the medications because all of the medication that was given to me only made the bleeding and clotting worst.

I had huge clots falling out of me and there was nothing that I could take to stop it. When I would go to the emergency room doctors thought that I was having a miscarriage because of the many clots that were falling out of me. My thought was maybe I was dying internally.

I would like to encourage you to stay strong and don't give up. Be encouraged and keep pressing through your pain and embarrassing moments. Be encouraged and know that some people pay a higher cost in life to be who they are don't allow this to break you but allow this to make you stronger and better. Everyone is dealing with some type of issue in their life it may not be in their health but we all have an issue or a deficiency that plagues us in some type of way. My prayers are that you don't allow your issues to have the last say so as to what the final outcome of your health shall be. Be encouraged and know that you are bigger then what you are up against and you have the power to fold or keep fighting. I would like to encourage you when you are feeling tired, hopeless, and depleted to hold on and believe that greater is coming. My prayers are that you don't view yourself as defeated but as a mighty warrior who won't stop until she has conquered her healing.

My prayers are that you don't allow fibroids to write the rest of the chapters of your life but that you take control and give the chapters a new life and a voice that says I am whole and no longer tormented. My prayers are that you allow your voice to speak louder than your attacks. My prayers are that as you continue to work through your issue of blood or fibroids that you maintain your joy in the process. My prayers are that you suffer no more and that your, tears, prayers and desires of your heart are answered. Be encouraged and run your race knowing that you are not alone.

Vaginal Discharge

This is another one of those topics that women are afraid to talk about not to say that I blame them because vaginal discharge is an unpleasant, irritating, and discomforting experience. My friends use to call me a hypochondriac. They would say that I would go to the doctor for anything and everything which wasn't true. I believe in listening to my body when it speaks. I also believe that it is better to be safe than to be sorry. I don't see any harm in getting a second opinion or even a third if necessary.

Whenever I would go to the doctor about my vaginal discharge I was always given medication for a yeast infection or for (BV) which is bacterial vaginosis. My cultures never came back showing that I had a STD or BV but I was always given Flagyl and Diflucan or a vaginal cream to take for the vaginal discharge. It wasn't until after I found out that I had fibroids that I also found out that having a vaginal discharge was common among women who had fibroids. I then began to take herbs, yeast guard, teas and Vitalzym but nothing worked. That is a short list of things that I had taken. The medication that the doctors prescribed only made the vaginal discharge worst. The natural products would work for a week or two but it didn't give me total relief from having a vaginal discharge. I also poured apple cider organic vinegar in my bath water which helped from time to time but if I used too much vinegar it would sometimes leave me feeling a little irritated. I didn't believe in taking douches because I believe that the body does cleanse itself; well at least that was my case. I found myself so desperate for some type of relief I tried taking an apple cider vinegar douche; let me tell you, it set my vagina on fire.

After my doctor looked over my test results which all came back negative my doctor didn't know what to say to me other than some women may experience having a light discharge which is natural and perfectly normal as long as it doesn't have a smell. I said to her this may be true, but that was not my normal. I knew that something was wrong because I still had a discharge. My doctor knew I wasn't prone to having yeast infections so she gave me a referral to go see a gynecologist who was a specialist. I went to see the specialist and he ordered an ample amount of testes to be ran and when those test results came back they were negative of any findings. The doctor stated that he couldn't find anything wrong with me and he didn't know why I was having a vaginal discharge other than it is natural for some woman to have. I didn't understand what was going on because I never used any fragrances below my waist and I always wore cotton panties.

Rather I wore panty liners or not I found myself being irritated. I even switched to wearing organic pads, panties, and panty liners; but that didn't work either. I stop eating meat, which is still something that I don't eat. I stop eating process foods and sugars. I stop using chemicals in my hair that wasn't organic. I also stop using chemicals on my body and clothes that wasn't organic. It didn't matter what I did or took nothing was giving me any relief as it pertained to my vaginal discharge. A lady that I knew suggested that I do acupuncture. I didn't know how that would help, but I didn't get around to doing acupuncture because I was so mentally and physically drained. I was too tired to try anything else; I was at my wits end. I was tired of all the suffering. I was glad about one thing, which was the vaginal discharge didn't have a smell.

There are some solutions that will come with side effects but you will have to weigh out your own pros and cons and do what works best for you. I wish I could say I found a solution or a resolution to resolving the problem for women who experience a vaginal discharge that is related to having fibroids. I wish I can say that I found a cure for fibroids; but the truth is I don't have an answer nor was I able to find an answer. I will say this, don't be so desperate to the point that you don't do the research on whatever you may consider taking. This experience for me was tormenting. When you go through an experience that attacks you physically and mentally at the same time; it makes the battle that much harder to fight and it intensifies the level of pain and suffering. When you have to fight for your mental and physical state of being it will leave you depleted and fatigued.

There were times where I couldn't think or feel anything; I just felt numb. After I added everyday life, work, money, kids, family, relationships, pets or anything else into the equation that was the recipe for a nervous breakdown.

I found myself overwhelmed and feeling like I was on a merry go round waiting for it to stop. There were many times I would find myself entangled in the busyness of life just so I wouldn't have to deal with my own personal suffering. It really is a miracle that I can write today in a sound mind without carrying all the weights and issues of fibroids or the issue of blood. I am grateful for a new beginning and I will stay hopeful that the resolution that I have chosen for me will work in my favor. I will continue to encourage other women while building and caring for my own personal health.

Beautiful Queens, Mothers, Daughters, Sisters, Aunts, Cousins, Ladies, Nieces, Grand-Daughters, Wives, and Women please take care of your body. While there is no for sure answer as to where fibroids come from; don't intentionally abuse your body with any unsafe practices that could cause your body harm. There are higher expectations and demands that are placed upon women. Our bodies tend to take a greater beaten then our male counterpart. Because women carry the weight and pain of child bearing, menopause and monthly cycles the female body really does goes through a lot. I am not suggesting that you go health crazy; nor am I indicating that what happens to your body is the direct cause of something that was done by you.

What I am saying is; because it is currently no known origin as to where the root of fibroids come from let's be more mindful of what we are putting in our bodies. Together we can partner in living a lifestyle that is healthy. I know this is hard for some women to practice due to certain barriers, but I believe that whatever effort that you put towards healthy living it will give you a better outcome of winning the battle on fibroids. By changing your habits my hopes are that women will see results that work. Also, I hope that you take the time to educate your daughter/s about fibroids and some of the issues that comes along with living with fibroids. I pray that one day the numbers will cease if not decrease of the many women who live with fibroids or the issue of blood.

Let's stand together so that fibroids can stop claiming the physical health and mindset of our women and daughters. Women all over the world are looking for answers; while we don't have an answer yet; my prayers are that you stay encouraged. My prayers are that you are healed and you will no longer have to deal with the issue of having a vaginal discharge or any other symptoms that is associated with having fibroids or the issue of blood. My prayers are that you walk in freedom in every area of your life and that you are free from all things that would cause you to suffer. Be encouraged.

The Womb

The uterus is the medical term for the womb. I want to talk about how most women feel about their womb. Many women have a strong attachment to their womb because the womb is the birthing place. Rather a woman wants a child or not she still wants to keep everything that she came into the world with. I know this to be true for most women because when a doctor says to a woman; I have to take your uterus a woman thinks about the detachment and being separated from her womb along with the thought of never being able to conceive or carry a child. At least that was my experience. Although, my tubes were tied, clipped and burned for 20 years when the doctor said to me I have to take your uterus, I gave him a weird look. I can't even tell you all the thoughts that were going through my mind in the 15 seconds that it took me to respond to the doctor. When I first asked the doctor about the process of having a hysterectomy I was quite shocked after hearing the process. The only thing that I was able to take way from the whole conversation of what the doctor said to me was uterus and you won't be able to have any more children.

Nevertheless, I still had an option of vitro fertilization if I wanted to have more children; but when the doctor said if he took my uterus I could never carry a child again I immediately said nope doc give me another solution. I felt like my emotions had been hit by a Mack truck because in the 15 seconds that it took me to respond I said to myself you won't be able to carry a child ever. The last thing that came across my mind was there won't be a procedure to reverse this if this is your choice. In my mind I felt like my choice and my rights had been stripped. After I was done analyzing the baby situation my thoughts were, am I going to feel empty inside or was I going to feel like I had stuff dangling around inside of me with no structural balance if I chose the hysterectomy.

All I heard the doctor say was when I take your uterus out no matter what you feel, think or want you will never be able to conceive or carry a child again. I also heard the doctor say you have a health problem and if you choose to have a hysterectomy you will never be able to have children again. The doctor didn't exactly say that to me that was my selective hearing moment. I felt like I was on trial standing in front of a judge and a jury and the case that was before the judge was; I have an issue that pertains to my health that was no fault of my own and no one has an answer as to where it came from and the sentence that was given to me was "Never to have kids, ever", the reason, because you have fibroids, so, your rights have been revoked and terminated, now go and live your life, however it may suit you; after this surgery.

I know that sounds harsh but you would be amazed of what your ears hear when something is being said to you that is not to your liken. On the other hand I looked at how fortunate I was because I was blessed to have two children before having to make such a hard decision. Then I thought about the many women who never had children but want children. I couldn't gain a positive thought or a good outcome from anything the doctor was saying to me after he gave me the option of having a hysterectomy. That was a hard pill to swallow but I knew that I had to make a choice about my situation because I truly couldn't take the pain and the bleeding anymore. I knew that I was tired of suffering and I had to decide what I was going to do without being in my emotions. I knew that I had to renew my mind if I wanted a different outcome. I knew that I had to speak differently because my confession was; this is my womb and nobody is going to take it, I have to protect my womb because it is a part of me and I will not let anything or no one take it from me rather she is sick or not. I considered my womb to have been sick because she was covered with fibroids. I left the doctor's office and did more research as to what would work best for me. It took me three more years of going through excruciating pain and suffering before I was able to make a choice of what I thought would be the best surgical procedure for me.

There is so much that could be said about the womb of a woman and the power that she possesses. I believe this is why so many women first reaction is an emotional reaction because she is being asked to detach from something that gives her the power to produce and enable's her to birth a child into the world. For most women the thought is hard to fathom. I had to ask myself, do you want to keep your womb and suffer with your current pain and condition;

or do you want to go through several surgical procedures risking further damage and still not resolve the initial problem; or is it worth having multiple surgeries verses having one surgery? It all boiled down to one question for me which was, did I want to keep my womb or not?

I know the power of the womb, but I also know the power of me as a person. My hopes and prayers are if you desire to have children I pray that you are able to conceive a child before you have to make the choice that could cost you your choice. Never give anything or anyone power over you as to how you should live your life. Never allow the criticism of others to affect your choice. Don't allow circumstances to predict the outcome of your health. Remember that you are stronger then what you are facing and don't allow fibroids or anything else to tell you that you are not.

My prayers are that you look at the deeper beauty that lives within. My prayers are that you don't allow child birthing to be the only thing that you birth but that you birth all that is within you. I am sure that you too have a book inside of you or poems that needs to be published or some type of dream or business that is waiting to be birth. Don't stop birthing because a doctor has suggested removal of your womb. Don't lose hope but keep pressing and keep birthing because you are a Giant and Giants don't easily fall. You are an Eagle and Eagles don't lower the quality of what they birth, they only soar higher. Beautiful Queens don't stop living or birthing because of one problem. Life is full of problems and you have to press through your problems and stumbling blocks. If you won all the other battles don't stop now reshuffle the deck and deal a hand that you can play; one that is most favorable for you. Be encouraged.

The Pain of it All

The pain of it all is what it has cost you to be you. It's all that you have endured along with the hidden pain that you suffer behind closed doors that only you know about. It's the pain that cause you to weep and travail in sorrow while you suffer alone. It's the pain that cause you to fall to your knees and say Lord why me. It's the pain that makes you sometimes wish that you wasn't born. It's the pain that plead for healing; but allows you to still suffer while you wait. It's the pain that cause life to be unbearable because you are such an emotional wreck. It's the pain that places limits on you and afflicts your mind, body, spirit and soul. It's the pain that troubles you and causes you to be despondent, upset, worried, depressed, angry, and bitter. It is the pain of it all.

One thing to remember about pain is when you are going through any type of pain no matter what type of pain or where it is rooted from; pain is pain and it all hurts. This experience of living with fibroids and the issue of blood have taken so much from me but it has also showed me how strong of a person, mother, daughter, wife, friend, minister, sister, and aunt that I am. Rather I was in pain or not I still had a role to fulfill where people needed or depended on me in-spite of my own personal pain. It wasn't like my role was eliminated until I was healed. Oftentimes I wished that it could've been but that was not the case. I still was expected to perform in my pain. Sometimes I found myself being out of breathe and bleeding like crazy and left with no energy or having the strength to do anything but I kept pushing myself because I knew others depended on me. The lesson that I learned was; when pain is suppressed it will show up at some point and time pending on your level of pain. You can only hide how you feel or what you are going through for a little while before the pain of it all shows up and reveal what you are really going through.

I remember there were times where I would wish and think myself to be whole and healed; then there were other times I could see myself healed but then the reality of the pain showed up and reminded me that I was still living in my pain and suffering. I didn't give up on my vision of seeing myself healed but there were so many times that I lost hope. I had days where I thought my healing was impossible because all signs pointed to a road of despair. I still kept holding on no matter how little my progress was.

I didn't stop believing but I had many days where the light was damn. I got tired of fighting and fighting alone. It's harder to fight when your vision is cloudy and your thought process has been hijacked; or when you have been in a battle for so long hoping, wishing, praying, standing, and believing for a change and nothing is working. I remember saying to myself this could be so much easier to deal with if I didn't have to carry it alone.

Sometimes you can be with someone and still feel like you are by yourself because the person with whom you are with isn't fully vested in the pain and suffering in which you are going through. Some women may have a partner or significant other with whom she is in a relationship with but that doesn't necessarily mean that she has the support, guidance and understanding that is needed while she is going through her storm. Not everyone gives mercy or grace to others in their time of need. Some people have been conditioned to take at the cost of someone else's pain or suffering. You will find out that people will want you to continue to serve them while you are in a broken, sick and weak state of being. Some people will still expect for you to perform as though nothing is wrong. Many women have been conditioned not to show pain but to bear pain even at a cost of hurting themselves. Women today are expected to give birth to a child and go back to work within six to eight weeks or less leaving no time for the body to properly heal. Women are also given the same time frame of six to eight weeks when they have a hysterectomy. This goes back to the conditioning of not to show pain even when you are in pain.

Many women have learned to produce in their suffering, brokenness and pain even if it cost them their life. One of the hardest decisions that women are faced with is when she has to make a decision about her health or her job. I have been faced with having to make this decision a few times and it is not easy. I had so many questions running through my mind as I am sure many women can relate to if you have ever been placed in a situation where you had to choose between your health or your job. It can seem like the ending of a nasty love affair or the beginning of a sweet first date. These are a few things that ran across my mind. Do I allow others to predict my coming or going, my health or healing, my pain and suffering, or my right to live a life that will bring healing and comfort? For every hurdle that a woman climbs she will encounter at least 3 more challenges that she will have to face in order to embrace the change in which she seeks. Rather her challenge is through a sacrifice, lack or a struggle she won't just arrive without knowing she had to pay a price. Every woman has her own pain of it all; but whatever your pain is don't allow fibroids or others to predict your outcome. Hold your head up high and repeat these words; this too shall pass. Be encouraged.

My prayers are that you suffer no more. My prayers are that you become a better, stronger and healthier you. My prayers are even-though your pain and suffering has cost you a lot; I pray that you don't lose hope and that you continue believing for your healing to come. My prayers are that you keep pressing through your pain. My prayers are that you don't allow anyone to stop you from improving your quality of life.

Nobody knows the battles that you fight when you are in a dark place. I am not talking about the picture that you paint for others to see; but the sweat, tears, and suffering that it has cost you to be who you are that nobody sees. I know the pain of living with fibroids and the issue of blood all too well and the associated cost that comes with it. I can attest to the pain of it all. Be encouraged and know that I feel your pain, maybe not to the level or exact depth in which you suffer, but I can identify with the pain that you feel and I pray for your healing in the Lord.

When you have done all that you know to do

What do you do when you have prayed, trusted, believed, taken medication, taken natural herbs, lost weight, changed your diet, tried meditation, and exercised? What do you do when you feel like you have done everything but still nothing works? What do you do when you don't have the strength to encourage yourself? What do you do when you stop believing for a cure that could bring healing to your situation? What do you do when you are the only one left standing in your fight and everyone else has abandoned you? What do you do when every door that you knock on gives you an answer of no or I can't? What do you do when you want to give up? I have one answer; it is; keep standing and keep believing and hoping for your healing. Never stop believing in you even when others do. Never stop believing for your healing no matter how many times that you are shamed. Always believe in you and for the best outcome even when your vision gets blurred. When you have done all that you can do the only thing left to do is stand.

I have learned to stand when I am being afflicted in my body, when I am in pain, when I am suffering, when I have tears rolling down my face, when I am broken, embarrassed, torn, being prosecuted, judged, shamed, made a fool of, going through the storms of life, bankrupt in my mind and body, when I have a little progress or when I have no progress; when others have lied on me, when I am not able to do for myself, when I am alone with no one to stand with me or when I am left standing in a puddle of blood.

I have learned to stand when I wanted to give up, when I felt like falling, when I didn't know where my next meal was going to come from, when I couldn't hear what to do or what direction to go in. I have learned to stand through the good times and the bad times. I have learned to stand through the rough and tough times, through all the times where I had no energy or strength to fight or get back up after I have fallen. I have learned to stand in the midst of my unbelief and when my mind was being tormented by my condition or situation. I have learned to stand when life dealt me a hand that I didn't ask for and when the odds were stacked against me. I have learned to stand when people have judged me by what statistics had to say instead of giving me an opportunity equal of someone else. I have learned to stand when things aren't in my favor and when all hell is breaking loose in my life. I have learned to stand through the abuse, failed marriages and relationships. I have learned to stand through the DUI's, dysfunctional upbringing, violent environment, having bad credit, having good credit and having vehicles repossessed. I have learned to stand even when I was homeless or jobless. I have learned to stand when I had no education to being educated. I have learned to stand when I had insurance to go to the doctor and when I didn't have any insurance. I have learned to stand without ever having a mentor and learning from the school of hard knocks. I have learned to stand even when I didn't want to stand and I wanted to give up. I have learned to stand with someone or alone; no matter the terms or the struggle I have learned to stand.

I have always told myself quitting is not an option. What does that means to me? I can have a time and moment to feel whatever type of way that I need to feel to relieve some pressure, stress or worries, but I can't live in a fallen state of mind where I don't get back up. I have trained my mind not to die in the broken places. No matter how long it may take me to get back up after a fall I press to stand towards a mark that is higher. When I learned how to stand from previous situations in my life I knew I couldn't let the issue of blood or fibroids keep me in an inoperable state.

Oftentimes I would evaluate certain moments in my life where I saw victory after the storm and those were the moments that would give me the energy to continue seeking healing while I was yet in my pain and suffering. Think about some of the stuff that you have made it through; no matter how you had to stand you are still here. I want to encourage you on all of your stands and say to you don't give up now. Continue to stand and don't quit; it's ok to take a breather or rest when needed, but don't quit. I know that there are times and days where it gets rough but don't stop living and don't stop seeking a resolution for your healing.

Nobody said life would be easy. In life, people are faced with barriers and obstacles that are challenging. Keep pressing until you get the result that says you win. Remember winning also has its pros and cons as well. You may win in one area but encounter other issues that may or may not be as extreme as the issues that you dealt with as it pertains to fibroids or the issue of blood. For every cause there is an effect and for every healing there still may be a slight defect; be grateful even in imperfections and through methods of faults or flaws that are not your own. Nothing is perfect; be thankful for the little things and be content in all things until your change comes.

Many of you have scars that you can see and some that are hidden. Wherever your scars are remember that those scars are taken from the one percent of imperfection; from a place in which we all have. Remember your scars are a reminder of your pain and suffering but it also represents what it has cost you to still be living and what it has cost you to stand. Remember that your scars were brought with a price and you are still standing in spite of the mark that was left. One thing you should remember about the scars are; they could have taken your life but they were left as a reminder as to what battles you had to fight and the end result was you didn't give up. Be encouraged and remember that some people will have bigger and more battles to fight then others; it doesn't mean that others won't have any battles to fight; it means that some things are out of our control.

My prayers are that as you endure your storm that you continue to stand. My prayers are that each day you grow stronger. I pray that your body is replenished daily with the proper amount of energy. I pray that your iron levels are balanced and your body lines up to a healthy place where you no longer experience lack. My prayers are that you grow wiser in the process of self-care, self-love and self-worth and that you use the tools and information that you gain to help you to be the best you possible. My prayers are that you continue to seek your healing and you are favored in the process of your healing. Be encouraged and continue to stand.

Surgery

I know throughout the entire book I didn't say exactly what I did about my fibroids. I sort of talked around my resolution about what I did when it came to me getting relief from dealing with fibroids and the issue of blood. Although, many of you might have guessed what my method of resolution was I will share with you what worked for me; again every woman has to make her own choice as to what will work for her. My choice was to get a hysterectomy; the procedure that was done was Davinci Hysterectomy and Bilateral Salpingectomy. The type of hysterectomy that my doctor and I decided on didn't require the removal of my ovaries. My doctor didn't want to remove my ovaries because he felt there wasn't a need to take them considering that I was only 43 years old. Also, my doctor didn't want to put me into early menopause by taking my ovaries if there wasn't a need to.

I by no means promote any woman to get a hysterectomy because just like anything else it to has its pros and cons. However, I will promote that you do what is best for you and be happy with whatever decision that you make. Nobody has to live your life but you. Every woman body is different and every woman overall health will be different. I am a healthy woman in spite of the issue that I dealt with that pertained to fibroids and the issue of blood. I was considered healthy enough to have my surgery with no complications because I wasn't over weight, I wasn't on any medications, I didn't have any prior health issues and I maintained a healthy diet. I am not saying that this has to be where you are in your health; I am sharing where I was in my health before having my surgery. I tried to avoid getting a hysterectomy like most women. I must admit I feared having such a major surgery; I wanted what I thought was the total make-up of a woman, which was my womb.

When I spoke to other women who were considering having a hysterectomy I found out that they had some of the same concerns as I did which were; I'm not going to be able to ever have children, I wonder is this going to affect my sex drive, I wonder am I going to experience vaginal dryness, I wonder if my husband or mate will view me as still being a whole woman, I wonder if I am going to be that woman who will experience complications after surgery or have issues while in surgery, I wonder will I have the help that will be needed while I am recovering. I wonder am I going to have a swollen belly like some women get after having a hysterectomy, I wonder if I am going to have problems urinating or problems with my bowel. I wonder how long will it take me to heal entirely, I wonder how this will affect me as a woman, I wonder what would other women think of me if they knew I had an hysterectomy, I wonder if this is going to be the right choice for me. Those same fears and concerns were running through my mind to the point where I didn't know if I was making the right choice or not.

Once I dealt with some of my I wonders, I then had to weigh my cost about everything and choose what would work best for me. Given very few options with none of them being to my liken I had to think about what I was currently going through and how much longer could I endure the pain and suffering. When I looked at the other procedures that I could have chosen; I realized that they all had their pros and cons. If I had gone with one of the other procedures there would have been a higher chance of the fibroids coming back. I knew whatever procedure I had chosen to go with, I only wanted to have one surgery. I didn't want to try all the other procedures and risk the fibroids coming back and having to have multiple surgeries.

Later I thought to myself why did I have such a major surgery done first? But then I thought; if I had tried one of the other procedures first, could I have been one of the few women where the fibroids didn't come back? Then the thought came across my mind, if I would have chosen one of the other procedures I would have been able to keep my uterus. The question then arose, how long would that last before the nightmare of fibroids returned back unto me? That is an answer that will remain unanswered because after counting up my cost having one surgery worked best for me.

When you have a hysterectomy, the chances of fibroids coming back are slim in comparison to having one of the other surgical procedures. Will a woman encounter other issues; for some women yes; while other women will experience minimal issues after having a hysterectomy. This is why you have to count up your own cost and do your research so that you can make the best choice. As I stated before having a hysterectomy is a major surgery for a woman. I know that some doctors and others would like to make it sound as easy and simple as 1-2-3, but it is not. The recovery time and other issues that some women may experience can be worst then their prior issues before having a hysterectomy. Today there are new and less invasive ways of doing hysterectomies than in times past, but it doesn't take away from the fact that having a hysterectomy is a major surgery.

Most doctors give women a time frame of six to eight weeks to heal after having a hysterectomy and then she is told that she can resume her regular activities in moderation pending if she feels ok. However, that may be the case for a small percentage of women but if women were to tell the truth about their true recovery time, it takes up to a year and for others they continue to have problems after having a hysterectomy. There are a lot of things that doctors won't be able to tell you about the recovery process because it will be different for every woman. Doctors are clueless about the many side effects that women encounter after having a hysterectomy. Doctors can only go by what they assume or by what research have been presented to them or what other women have shared about their personal experience.

There are many side effects to what is offered as a cure but what is important is that you weigh your current situation with what is being offered and be comfortable with accepting what the new cure may cost you. I can't stress enough, please be proactive in your research and also finding the best doctor who has experience in doing whatever procedure that you choose. My prayers are that as I walk in my healing that you too shall walk in the fullness of your healing. My prayers are as I continue to believe and hope for the best result in my recovery, I hope that you don't lose hope in believing that you can be healed.

Be encouraged and always remember that you have to be your number one cheerleader even if everyone else stops cheering. Be encouraged no matter what you are faced with. No woman wants to have a hysterectomy knowing that it can cause other issues down the line; but when your hands are forced and you are pressed then you have to do what is necessary. Life is filled with so many choices good and not so good. I believe that whatever chance that you are given to live a better quality of life then what you had you should grab hold of it and make the best out of a bad situation.

Women we are powerful, strong, beautiful, unique, creative, gifted and talented, let's make the choice to live and not die in lost hope, let's be positive role models for other women and young women who have fallen short or who lack the strength to complete her journey. Let's pour our whole self into one another. Please remember that a healthy recovery is just as important as the actual surgery; it all goes hand and hand. My prayers are that women all over the world be healed from the issue of blood and fibroids. I pray that women are no longer afflicted in their bodies. I pray that women began to experience a healthier lifestyle. I pray that as women and young women walk together this thing called fibroids will no longer be an epidemic that continues to attack women. Be encouraged.

All is Well

The beast is gone and I have been giving a second chance to live life without the issue of blood or fibroids. Everything in life is a process I am grateful to live one day at a time with hopes that I have been given a better quality of life. This has been a long journey but I thank God for the strength to endure. When I speak to others about my experience of living with fibroids and the issue of blood many people say, there is no way that I could have endured that. My response is; if you are given no other choice then you will do what you have to do. The easiest thing to do is to give up. I can give up on somethings; but I can't give up on me.

I have had people to walk out of my life, abandon me, and others who have left me feeling naked and ashamed; which has taught me to be my number one supporter. I have learned through my pains and sufferings how to stand even when I don't want to, even when I am in doubt, even when I lose the strength to press toward my mark, even when I lose the courage and hope to move on. I have learned to get back up even in my shame. I am a trained fighter but it is only through my battles that I have learned how to press and fight; it is through my pains and sorrows where I have won my biggest fights, it is through my hurts and difficult moments where I have learned to forgive and love me and others in spite of what was sown. The battles and the many scars that I possess has taught me not to hide my wounds or cover them up but to expose them so that others who may be going through some of the same battles can be encouraged while they are going through there storm.

I have entered into an agreement and become one with the statement; "All is well" even when it doesn't look well, because I know that my life won't always be filled with such great pain and suffering and even if it is; I will use it to help bring healing to others. I have learned that my life is not my own and it has been brought with a price so however the Lord choose to use it, I will remain an open vessel for Him to do so. It is through my life and hardships the Lord will breathe life into the lives of others. It is through my life that others shall see the works that the Lord has done and continues to do. It is through my life and testimonies the Lord will bring healing, strength, and empowerment to others. It is through my life that has been openly exposed; that others will be set free and released from the yoke of bondage.

Everything in life has purpose and we may not know the purpose behind all the things that happens in our life but be assured that it is preparing you for something and building something in you. It is molding you to be the best you possible. One thing that I have learned about training is; Father Yahweh trains differently than the way that man trains. His ways are truly not our ways that is for sure. I know many of you can look back over your life and say wow, I went through somethings that should have killed me; but I am still standing; others may be able to say I have a limp from the many battles that I have fought but I am still standing. It is something about the stand that gives a person the power to continue to walk even when they feel like giving up. There will be obstacles, storms, trails, situations, circumstances, testes and barriers that we all will have to face one day. What matters the most is that you recognize that this is a part of life and you don't give up.

There shouldn't be a question as to if we will be faced with challenges the true question is when. In life you have a choice to be bitter about what you go through or you can make the choice to learn from what happened in your life and use it in a positive manner to be a better person rather than a bitter person. Food for thought, if you allow everything that you go through in life to make you bitter and angry then you will never experience any peace or joy in your life. When you choose to be bitter your life will be filled with hurt and you will speak from a place of pain. Don't allow the issue of blood or fibroids to tell you what you can't have. Don't feel sorry for yourself because of the choice that you had to make about having a hysterectomy or any other surgical procedure that you may have to have. Always remember that you are a whole woman in spite of what you think, feel, or believe; free yourself and live again.

I have seen marriages and relationships be destroyed because of women having to make the choice to have a hysterectomy, my question is why? People see you how you see yourself. I ask that you see yourself whole and complete. Being able to have a baby isn't the only thing that makes up the DNA and characteristic of being a woman, yes that is the desire of many women but you shouldn't allow that to define who you are? You have to have a strong mindset and take authority over your thoughts and who you are as a person. You are bigger then what comes up against you. If anybody leaves you because of a choice that you had to make in order that you may have a better quality of life than they were not for you.

Women go through a lot mentally and physically but you have to take care of you because who will if you don't. Once you are done taking care of everything and everybody else who is seeing about you? Once the kids, husband, partner, the dog, cat, family, friends, bills, and the house, is taking care of, who sees about you? One fact to remember is; if you are not in your best state mentally, spiritually, emotionally and physically; then what are you really given in terms of seeing about everybody else and never taking the time to care for you? I will tell you, broken and fragmented pieces of you. You have to allow others to be accountable when it comes to assisting you when you are in need. In life you will find people who take and others, who give, don't allow others to take when you don't have much to take and your tank is already running on empty. Don't continue to hurt yourself at the cost of someone else who is being insensitive to your needs.

With that being said, I would like to encourage women all over the world to keep pressing through your pain and suffering; I know that every women situation is different, but I believe the end result for us all is to be healed. Nobody said that this thing called life would be a walk in a park but together we can hit a home run and shoot for as many wins as possible. Together let's change the way that we view ourselves and our thought process as a woman, mother, queen and daughter. Let's give ourselves a higher level of value and worth regardless of what we go through. One of my prayers are; Lord don't let me look like what I am going through or what I have been through. People would always look at me when I say that until I share a couple of my war stories with them and that's when they would be in awe about all that the Lord has done in me and through me. That is also my prayer for every woman across the globe.

I pray that you are given the recovery time necessary for your healing. My prayers are that every woman be mighty in their purpose and destiny in which they were created. My prayers are that women all over the world come together in unity and birth daughters that have the wisdom of God. My prayers are that women learn to be a midwife for other women in their time of need. My prayers are that women intercede in prayer for other women to be healed and restored. My prayers are; everyone who reads this book spreads knowledge to others who are unaware about what some women go through who has fibroids or who lives with the issue of blood. Be encouraged.

My Prayers to You

I declare and decree that this book reaches and touches the lives of women all over the world and impacts the minds and hearts of women who are suffering with fibroids or the issue of blood. I declare and decree that women stop living in shame about fibroids. I declare and decree that women start support groups that will bring healing to other women who have fibroids or the issue of blood. I declare and decree that all women be free from sickness. I declare and decree that all women walk in the joy and peace that the Lord gives. I declare and decree that all woman stand together until unity and true sisterhood is formed. I declare and decree that the love of God will fill the hearts of women and cover them while they are in their process of healing. I declare and decree that a hedge of protection is placed over and around you and no weapons that form against you shall prosper. I declare and decree that every woman who has fibroids or the issue of blood no longer live in isolation, shame, fear, anger, or humiliation. I declare and decree that you will no longer feel helpless, depressed, emotional, or abandoned. I declare and decree that the Lord hears your cry and that you no longer deal with the issue of being anemic. I declare and degree that the beast no longer lives within and that you no longer deal with the issue of having a vaginal discharge. I declare and degree that your womb be restored and made healthy. I declare and decree that your pain of it all cause you to stand and not fall. I declare and decree that when you have done all that you know to do that you stand and don't give up. I declare and decree that your surgical procedure is a success. I declare and decree that All is well. I declare and decree that you suffer no more and all pain is removed from your body. I declare and decree that sickness is removed from your body. I declare and decree that All things are working together for your good. I declare and decree that the Lord favors you and grants you health insurance or the resources to see about your health. I declare and decree that the Lord keep your mind in all that you go through. I declare and decree that your mind be renewed and that you are no longer tormented by the pain and agony of living with fibroids or the issue of blood. I declare and decree that you have the help and assistance that is needed as you walk out your process. I declare and decree that blood will no longer be an issue or the smell of blood. I declare and decree that your faith to believe is strengthen and you walk in victory. I declare and decree that you are given a second chance and you live a life that is healthy, fruitful and productive. I prophesy that you walk in your purpose and destiny in which you were created. I prophesy that every woman walks as a proverbs 31 woman. I prophesy that every area in your life be healed. I prophesy that women all over the world birth all that is within them. I prophesy that there will not be any premature death over your life. I prophesy that you will live and not die. I prophesy that your visions and dreams will no longer remain dormant. I prophesy that every lie that the enemy has spoken to you that it be cursed and sent to the pits of hell never to return back unto you. I prophesy that every unclean spirit that has attached itself to you die and be sent to the pits of hell and never return unto you. I prophesy that you be made whole and you suffer no more. I loose the Favor of the Lord over your life; I loose His wisdom, joy, peace, and love over your mind body spirit and soul. I bind and loose every stronghold that would try to hold you back from the will and purpose and plan of the Lord off your life. I plead the blood of Jesus over your mind, body, spirit and soul. I plead the blood of Jesus over your monies, your home, your health, and all that is a part of your destiny. I plead the blood of Jesus over these prayers and that He will hear the cries of His Daughters and He will answer these prayers and the tears of your pain and sorrow. I pray that these prayers are covered in the Blood; in Jesus mighty name. Amen

www.ingramcontent.com/pod-product-compliance
Lightning Source LLC
Chambersburg PA
CBHW050543300426
44113CB00012B/2234